HOW TO FREE YOURSELF FROM PAIN

TREATMENT FOR MANY COMMON AILMENTS
FROM HEADACHES TO LOWER BACK PAIN
BY USING ACUPRESSURE, THERMAL THERAPY, DIET
THERAPY, AND HERBAL THERAPY USING GINSENG

By Dr. Pedro Chan

PRICE/STERN/SLOAN
Publishers, Inc., Los Angeles
1982

Copyright ©1982 by Pedro Chan
Published by Price/Stern/Sloan Publishers, Inc.
410 North La Cienega Boulevard, Los Angeles, California 90048

Printed in the United States of America. All rights reserved. No part of this
publication may be reproduced, stored in a retrieval system, or transmitted,
in any form or by any means, electronic, mechanical, photocopying, record-
ing,·or otherwise, without the prior written permission of the publishers.

ISBN: 0-8431-0347-7

LIBRARY OF CONGRESS CATALOG CARD NUMBER: 81-85643

This book is dedicated to the medical professionals and to those millions of patients who have benefited from acupuncture and acupressure.

THE BEGINNING

"Nothing should be omitted in an art which interests the whole world, one which may be beneficial to suffering humanity and which does not risk human life or comfort."

–Hippocrates

TABLE OF CONTENTS

PAIN RELIEF STARTS WITH YOU

The Only Pain That Is Easy to Bear
Is the Pain of Others

There are not many conditions that qualify as being truly universal. Pain is one of the few that knows no boundaries. In degree, pain varies from the little prick of a finger that elicits a mild "Ouch!" through headaches and muscle pulls that bring forth moans and groans of discomfort, to the disabling traumas that result in screams of anguish.

Pain strikes us all. It cares not about geographical or national borders, politics, skin color, religion, or time of day. From the first slap on the backside that sparks the reaction of breath and a cry announcing our birth to the final moment of life before death takes over, we all experience pain.

In spite of the universal familiarity every person has with pain, it is one of the most elusive things to define. Webster's Collegiate Dictionary defines pain as "An affection or feeling proceeding from a derangement of functions, disease, or bodily injury." Take note: Webster's says a "feeling." It does not say what kind of feeling. Certainly it is not a feeling that makes us laugh but just the opposite.

Webster's has our sympathy; pain is a most difficult word to define. If one takes to the streets and asks 20 people to describe pain, one gets back 20 different descriptions. Pain can only be described in the light of experience, and then only to one's self. It is nearly impossible to detail one's experience of pain so that it can be sensed or understood by another who has not had the same experience.

If a person says to you, "It hurt just as if I had hit my finger with a hammer," that is a graphic description. But if you have never hit your finger with a hammer you have no way of knowing that feeling. You lack the experience to sense that feeling of pain. However, if someone says, "It hurt just as if I had stubbed a toe," and in the past, you have stubbed your toe, you can identify with that feeling and know precisely what is meant.

From the above it is obvious that pain is a very personal feeling. There are, however, wide variances in the tolerance people have for pain. What is excruciating for one may be only a minor ache for another whose threshold of pain is much higher. With this in mind, it's easy to understand how the latter person might belittle the suffering of the first and cause even more anguish through an unsympathetic attitude. When one is in pain, one wants relief, not to be told his suffering is insignificant.

The Pain Problems and Solutions

An estimated 8 to 10 precent of the population suffers from some form of migraine headache. Arthritis alone afflicts over 50 million Americans, 20 million of whom require medical care. Each year arthritis claims 600,000 new victims and its cost to the national economy is estimated to be nearly $13 billion. Lower back pain, another of the most common pain complaints, had totally disabled seven million Americans, and according to the National Center for Health Statistics, generates nearly 19 million visits to doctors annually. Add to these the many other pain-related disordes – facial and dental pain, neuralgia, etc. – and it is understandable how chronic pain can cost the nation an estimated $50 billion annually. Its cost in terms of human suffering and lost potential is incalculable.

Fortunately, for most of us pain is a temporary thing. It briefly comes and goes with illnesses and dysfunctions, yet rare indeed is the day when each of us does not experience some small pain.

Unfortunately, there are those who endure constant pain. They suffer a chronic condition that subjects them to a steady attack. The presence of pain is the norm for these hapless numbers and they are often driven to the overuse of drugs and other chemical remedies that can become pervasive and end up adding to the problem rather than alleviating it.

The individual who suffers chronic pain seeks relief as a matter of survival. It becomes essential that some method of easing the pain be found. Often the unchecked pain causes its sufferer to seek all manners of strange remedies and to act in bizarre ways, without benefit.

Many new pain-killing drugs have been developed and are constantly touted as the final answer to pain. Electrical stimulation and surgery are sometimes implemented to stop pain, and acupuncture/acupressure is receiving more and more attention from medical experts throughout the world as a means of eliminating or reducing pain.

Any of these methods can have a place in the treatment of specific problems. But the single fact that applies to every victim of pain has already been stated here: pain is a very personal thing. As such, it must always be dealt with on a personal basis and it is the individual who must take the first step to be free of pain. What follows here is intended to serve as a guide through the process of self-treatment. This includes acupressure, moxibustion, auricular therapy, diet therapy, and herbal medicine using ginseng.

ACUPRESSURE THERAPY

Why Acupuncture/Acupressure?

Recent clinical trials at UCLA and other medical centers have demonstrated that acupuncture/acupressure can be helpful in the management of many chronic complaints that have not responded successfully to Western medical therapy. For example, in the treatment of intractable chronic pain, acupuncture/acupressure provides a therapeutic alternative which is often superior to drugs and surgery. Long-term use of analgesic agents can produce undesirable side effects and can lead to the development of tolerance. In addition, acupuncture/acupressure has been found to be extremely safe, effective, and free from serious side effects.

Acupuncture VS. Acupressure

Acupuncture is stimulation by the insertion of needles. Acupressure is stimulation by finger pressure. Both stimulations serve to prevent or modify the perception of pain, to normalize physiological functions including pain control, and to treat certain diseases or functions of the body. Acupuncture is invasive while acupressure is non-invasive. In most cases, acupressure may be slower and require more repetitions, but it is free, simple, easy-to-apply, and effective. It can be used anywhere and by anyone, without special medical knowledge. Subjects will not be frightened because there are no needle insertions. No equipment or drugs are needed in the procedure.

> *Acupressure is not intended to provide a substitute for acupuncture or conventional therapy. Acupressure should be used only as a supplement. For any conditions requiring medical treatment(s) see a licensed acupuncturist or physician.*

Acupressure Works

Reports from China indicate that acupressure does work. The First Medical College of PLA reported that extractions of teeth with finger pressure were performed on 3,444 cases with a success rate of analgesia in 97.8% cases and excellent or good results in 89%. Tonsillectomy and Maxillary Sinus operations with finger pressure were performed on 976 cases with a success rate of 99.2% and with an excellent or good analgesia rate of 90.1%. Subtotal Thyroidectomy with finger pressure was performed on 65 cases with a success rate of 96.9% and with an excellent or good analgesia rate of 89.2%. Subtotal Gastrectomy was also performed on 175 cases with a success rate of 90.2% and with an excellent or good analgesia rate of 72.6% The basic maniuplation of finger pressure was done by pressing before the operation and with firm massage during the operation.

It has been observed that when some points are stimulated by pressure for a certain length of time, the wave of the EEG will intensify and the theta waves will become more numerous. This fact suggests that the afferent impulses evoked by finger pressure have some inhibitory effect on the cerebrum. This seems to verify the recent discovery of endorphin release as a result of stimulating the acupuncture points. Many scientists and investigators have turned up evidence that stimulating some acupuncture points prompts the brain to release endorphins – perhaps from the pituitary or limbic system – which will then circulate as hormones and block pain pathways.

THERMAL (MOXA) THERAPY

More Than Acupuncture/Acupressure

The Chinese meaning of acupuncture is twofold: needles and moxibustion. Therefore, acupuncture/acupressure and moxibustion can be used together or individually for treatment.

Moxibustion is a form of thermal therapy applied near the acupuncture point. It is non-invasive and it is another form of self-treatment.

How To Do It

The thermal souce is provided by the burning of dry Chinese wormwood leaves (Artemis Vulgaris). It has the properties of warming, removing obstruction of the channels, and promoting the functions of the organs.

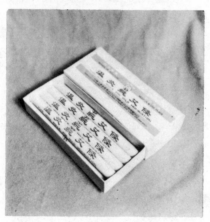

Moxa Rolls

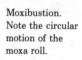

Moxibustion.
Note the circular
motion of the
moxa roll.

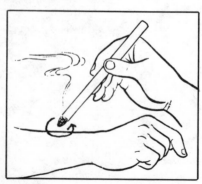

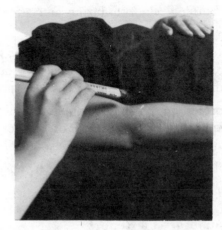

Moxibustion
over the elbow.

For external, indirect moxibustion, a moxa roll is always used. One end is ignited and place about one half to one inch away from the specific point. Move the roll over the point in a circular motion so the heat will not concentrate in one spot and burn the skin. If it gets too hot, simply move the roll a little further from the skin.

You usually apply warmth over each point for about 1-2 minutes, or until you see the local area becoming pink. Meanwhile you should feel a tingling sensation around that point. When that happens, it indicates that you are responding to the treatment.

Many of my patients complained that they had failed to respond to some form of thermal therapy (i.e. heating pad, hot shower, ultraviolet rays, etc.) before coming to my office. After moxibustion, they could feel a difference. That difference is the relief of pain.

Moxa heat has a short wave length which enables it to penetrate deep into the muscle tissues and stimulate the acupuncture point. Most thermal treatments provide superficial warmth only.

The effects of moxibustion are many: dilation of blood vessels, stimulation of blood circulation, and acceleration of metabolism. The patient always experiences a sense of complete relaxation and soothing comfort during and after the process of moxibustion.

A word of caution: do not use moxibustion on patients with high blood pressure or fever, hyperactivity, areas of acute inflammation (local redness), or on any area above the neck.

Moxibustion is performed on the same acupuncture points discussed in "Clinical Applications of Specific Pain Problems." Moxibustion points will be indicated for each case or point.

You can get moxa rolls from your local herb store. If you have difficulty finding them, please contact the author.

Case Study: An Acupuncturist's Report

I hurt my lower back twice last year. Each time it was sprained carrying heavy baggage or furniture. Instead of using needles or pressure, I used moxibustion on my lower back and lower extremities. The first treatment relieved my movement and some pain. A total of two treatments gave me complete relief within two days.

Many people asked me why I did not use needles since I am an acupuncturist. First, it would have been impractical to use acupuncture since I would not have been able to get a clear view of my back. Second, I did not apply pressure because I was in pain, and it was just too much to exert any kind of pressure at all.

You may say that as this was simply a sprain, I would have gotten well anyway, without any treatment. In my case the moxibustion helped to speed up the healing process by reducing the stiffness and suffering. At least instead of waiting for the slow relief, I was able to move around immediately after the moxibustion.

AURICULAR (EAR) THERAPY

Why The Ear?

Auricular therapy is similar to acupressure. However, instead of working on the body surface, we massage one or more specific points on the surface of the auricle (ear).

Most of us are aware that the ear is the organ of hearing as well as the center for controlling equillibrium. Few of us know that the ear represents a complete system of healing.

Anatomists divide the ear into three areas: (1) the external; (2) the middle; and (3) the inner ear. The external ear includes the auricle and the external meatus (the ear canal). This is the part of the ear that we are interested in studying in this chapter.

Currently, there are more than 200 points which have been discovered in the ear. This is mainly the result of accumulated research and clinical work in China during the past 20 years.

There are at least four major applications of auricular therapy: (1) preventive medicine, (2) therapy, (3) diagnostic aid, and (4) surgical analgesia. This chapter discusses mainly the therapeutic aspects of the ear and its use by the layman.

Auricular therapy can treat as many disorders as body acupuncture/acupressure can. In the many thousands of cases treated by auricular therapy in China, effectiveness has proved to be 70-80%. In many cases, it has even proven to be over 90% effective.

Treatment of pain problems by auricular therapy has also proved effective. It is especially good for pain from sprains, inflammation, neuralgia, arthritis, etc. In a study at the University Hospital Pain Clinic, London, Canada, auricular therapy was used on 27 patients with various pain problems. Results indicated that relief of pain was immediate in 25 patients (almost 93 percent). For some patients, pain was completely abolished; others reported modifications of pain.

In another study by Dr. Sai-il Chun of the Unversity of Pennsylvania, of 46 cases with 57 chronic pain syndromes of various nature, the success rate was 84% with an average of seven treatments. Problems ranged from trigeminal neuralgia, shoulder pain, tennis elbow, arthritis, lower back pain and headaches, to phantom pain, etc.

Universal Point For Pain Treatment

The "Shen-men" point is excellent for relief of pain and inflammation. Whenever and wherever there is body pain, the point will become sensitive. By sensitive, I mean that the "Shen-men" point is tender or causes discomfort when touched or pressed.

Point: *Shen-Men, meaning "Gods Gate" or "Divine Gate."*

Location: At the meeting of the lower and upper limbs of the antihelix. *(see diagram)*

Technique: Use the nail of the index finger to press down, then massage in a static, circular movement for about five seconds. Put your thumb behind the ear to aid the massage. Do not scratch the skin surface, it is very easy to break the skin if you do so. When you stimulate the point properly, you should feel some stinging heating sensation radiating from the point being massaged. First massage the ear on the affected side of the pain; if this fails, try the other side.

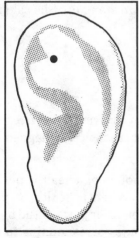

"Shen-men" point located at the meeting point of the lower and upper limbs of the anti-helix.

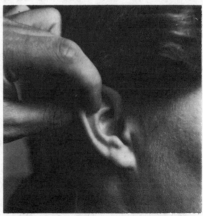

Massaging the "Shen-men" point with the nail of the index finger.

21

Remarks

This is the principal point for releif of any pain, especially pain with no known origins or etiology. In addition, "Shen-men" is also effective in the treatment of inflammation because of its properties in dirving off the heat and counteracting poison. In most cases pain is accompanied by inflammation. Therefore, "Shen-men" is one of the ideal points for such treatment. "Shen-men" can also induce relaxation because it calms the heart and the mind.

Case Study

Once, while attending a lecture, I sat next to a woman in her fifties who complained of lower back pain. I explained I might be able to help her if she would allow me to. I did not tell her I was an acupuncturist but she gave me her consent. Normally, I would start a lower back patient with some local points. Since I did not know her I chose not to treat her back directly, but decided to work on the ear closest to me. My efforts did not seem to have any effect. I then massaged the other ear, and immediately the woman said there was a funny sensation rushing to her lower back. I asked her to stand up. She said the pain was gone.

Organization of the Ear

The ear is made up of a layer of skin covering a thin irregular plate structure of elastic cartilage. There is no cartilage in the lobe.

Under normal conditions, the ear points of a healthy person do not have any special responses. When a health or pain problem exists in the internal organs or other parts of the body, there are one or more responsive points corresponding to the disorder. The degree of sensitivity at the point is directly proportional to the intensity of the illness.

The points can ony reflect the areas and organs of the disorder; they do not indicate the cause of the disorder. A Chinese study reported that a fracture of the leg in monkeys or rabbits causes some points to respond in the ear's triangular fossa and antihelix. These two areas of the ear correspond to pain in the leg area.

In another study of 288 tuberculosis patients in one hospital, 286 showed responses to a point in the "Lung" area of the ear.

Therefore, in addition to using the "Shen-men" point for general pain, corresponding points should be used. For example, if pain is in the elbow, add ear point "Elbow"; if pain is in the lower back, add ear point "Lower Back" or "Buttock," wherever it is more sensitive.

Descriptively, the ear is thought to represent an inverted fetus. *(Courtesy of Chan's Corp.)*

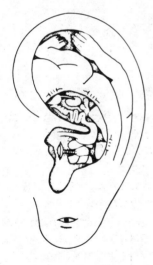

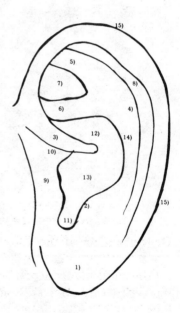

Distribution of ear points. *(Courtesy of Chan's Corp.)*

1. LOBE
2. ANTITRAGUS
3. HELIX LIMB
4. ANTIHELIX
5. UPPER LIMB OF ANTIHELIX
6. LOWER LIMB OF ANTIHELIX
7. TRIANGULAR FOSSA
8. SCAPHA
9. TRAGUS
10. SUPRATRAGIC NOTCH
11. INTERTRAGIC NOTCH
12. CYMBA CONCHA
13. CAVUM CONCHA
14. CONCHA EDGE OF ANTIHELIX
15. HELIX

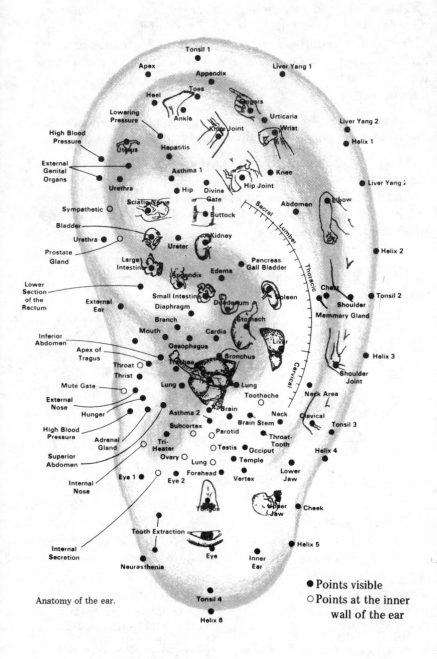

Anatomy of the ear.

- Points visible
- Points at the inner wall of the ear

24

The following is a list of anatomical parts of the ear and their relationship with the rest of the body:

1. **LOBE**
   Anatomy: Lower portion of the ear.
   Corresponds to: Facial region.

2. **ANTITRAGUS**
   Anatomy: An elevation above the lobe.
   Corresponds to: Head region .

3. **HELIX LIMB—**
   Anatomy: Transverse portion of helix extending into concha.
   Corresponds to: Diaphragm. Region around the helix limb corresponds to digestive tract.

4. **ANTIHELIX—**
   Anatomy: Curved ridge in front of helix.
   Corresponds to: Trunk.

5. **UPPER LIMB OF ANTIHELIX—**
   Anatomy: Upward branch of antihelix.
   Corresponds to: Lower extremities.

6. **LOWER LIMB OF ANTIHELIX—**
   Anatomy: Downward branch of antihelix.
   Corresponds to: Buttocks.

7. **TRIANGULAR FOSSA—**
   Anatomy: Triangular depression between upper and lower limbs of antihelix.
   Corresponds to: Genital organs.

8. **SCAPHA—**
   Anatomy: Bow-shaped groove between helix and antihelix.
   Corresponds to: Upper extremeties.

9. **TRAGUS—**
   Anatomy: The fleshy protrusion in front of the ear.
   Corresponds to: Adrenal gland and others.

10. **SUPRATRAGIC NOTCH—**
    Anatomy: Depressed part between upper tragus and limb of helix.
    Corresponds to: None

11. INTERTRAGIC NOTCH—
Anatomy: In depression between lower tragus and antitragus.
Corresponds to: Internal secretion.

12. CYMBA CONCHA—
Anatomy: Portion of concha above limb of helix.
Corresponds to: Abdominal region and organs there.

13. CAVUM CONCHA—
Anatomy: Portion of concha below limb of helix.
Corresponds to: Chest region and organs there.

14. CONCHA EDGE OF ANTIHELIX—
Anatomy: Curved edge of the antihelix with concha.
Corresponds to: Spinal column.

15. HELIX—
Anatomy: Outer curved rim of the ear.
Corresponds to: None.

16. BACK OF THE EAR—
Anatomy: At the back of the ear.
Corresponds to: Back region of fetus.

Case Study

On one occasion, I was demonstrating acupressure on a patient in one of my workshops in Florida. The patient had a shoulder pain with limited mobility. I started with body points, one by one, ranging from local points to distal points in the upper extremity and then the lower extremity. But there was no relief for the patient. Finally, I decided to try the "Shoulder Point" on the ear of the affected side. I used a retracted pen to do the massage. Again no relief. I was disappointed. And then with little expectation, I worked on the same point of the other ear. To my surprise, it worked. The patient raised her arm with almost complete freedom. The pain was substantially reduced.

Now, I always recommend that before you give up, try both ears, one by one. You never know which one is going to work for you until you have tried both of them.

DIET THERAPY

Why you Got a Headache

Have you ever wondered why you got a headache after eating some canned food or Chinese food? It is very simple. It is because monosodium glutamate (MSG) is added. Most canned foods contain MSG and some Chinese restaurants put MSG in the food to enhance the flavor. About five percent of the adult population will have reactions such as headache, nausea, or vomiting after ingesting MSG.

It is true that we are what we eat. "Food can feed you pain," says Dr. Neal Olshan, Director of the Pain Control Unit of the Mesa Lutheran Hospital in Scottsdale, Arizona. Dr. Olshan reported that up to 30% of all the pain people suffer, comes from the painful six: (1) monosodium glutamate; (2) Nitrites; (3) caffeine; (4) alcohol; (5) nicotine; and (6) tyramine. By avoiding the above items in your diet you may be able to reduce or even eliminate your pain or discomfort.

The Chinese emphasize the very important role diet plays in treating any kind of problem, especially pain problems. What you should eat is not as important as what you should *not* eat.

I find that many pain patients react to the ingestion of certain foods. These foods prolong pain suffering. It is imperative to *avoid* eating the foods described here.

Avoid Anything that Tastes Sour

Avoid anything that tastes sour, for example: vinegar; pickles; salad dressings; and all kinds of fruits, especially pineapples, lemons, oranges, mangoes, grapefruits, and other citrus fruits.

About eight years ago, I had a patient with trigeminal pain. After six acupuncture treatments, she still complained of the pain. At the last treatment, I asked her if she had been faithfully following my instructions by staying away from the above sour foods. She said yes. I then asked her to write down what she had eaten that day. At that point she recalled that she had been having a glass of lemonade every morning of her life. Because this was something she did all the time, she was not aware of it. She quit drinking the lemonade and with it went the pain. No further treatment was needed.

Avoid Cold or Icy Foods

Avoid cold or icy foods, for example: ice water; ice tea; ice cream; or any drink "on the rocks". Ingestion of cold or icy foods may cause constriction or restriction of blood circulation, which further induces discomfort if you have a pain problem.

I normally like to recommend that patients eat something light and warm (preferrably soup) before and after a treatment. Many times after treatment, a patient will go to a coffee shop and from there call to complain that the pain is worse than before. If no food was eaten, I ask the patient if he or she drank the ice water served. Usually the reply is, "Yes." That is why the pain is worse. Many times when you go to a restaurant you are automatically served ice water, and without hesitation you drink it. People don't pay attention to such small things, and yet small things such as this can hurt.

Avoid Alcoholic Beverages

Alcohol as a sedative drug may block the stimulation we try to generate for the treatment. Unfortunately, when you ask your patients to stop drinking, they often stop seeing you.

Avoid Spicy or Irritating Foods

Avoid spicy or irritating foods, for example: pepper; spices; chili sauces; etc. Eating these irritating items can cause pain to return after a patient's apparent recovery. Fortunately, this happens to only a small percentage of the patient population.

Cut Down Saturated Fats

It is important to cut down on the consumption of meats, such as beef and pork, that are high in saturated fats.

In Conclusion

You may wonder how long you have to stay away from the above foods. My answer is: For as long as you are getting treatment or as long as you continue to have the pain problem.

If at anytime after you are well you again feel pain, you should immediately trace what you ate the day before the pain began. You will see patterns emerging. You may find you are allergic to certain items. When you find out what they are, stay away from them forever.

My friend Dr. Collin Dong, author of two bestsellers, - *Arthritic's Cookbook* and *New Hope for the Arthritic* – is an excellent example of one who has used diet to help his own arthritis problem. At the age of 35, Dr. Dong was afflicted with a baffling form of arthritis that became progressively worse. Despite treatment by many specialists he was still helpless. He became so badly crippled he had to close down his medical clinic and retire at an early age. Experimenting with nutrition and diet, Dr. Dong finally brought about a dramatic change in his health. He is now in his seventies, free from pain and active in his practice specializing in the treatment of arthritic patients.

HERBAL THERAPY USING GINSENG

How to Detoxify the System

In our modern society, taking drugs of some kind is common-place. For example, the public consumes about 20 tons of asprin each day. Drugs have many side effects, though. For instance, some block the normal function of the pituitary glands. To detoxify the system and to restore the natural, healing powers of the body, I recommend taking "Panax Ginseng." Panax Ginseng is not just any common ginseng. You should be able to find Panax Ginseng in your local health food store, If not, write to the author.

I prefer to use the concentrated liquid. Use of the capsules, tea bags, or powders is not recommended for this kind of therapy. Take 5 c.c. of the concentrated ginseng daily for at least two weeks, or take the recommended quantity according to the label directions. I recommend taking it on an empty stomach. After taking it, do not ingest any food for two hours. You may drink some lukewarm water with it. This will help the ginseng work better.

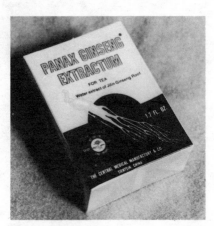

Panax Ginseng™ Extractum from the People's Republic of China.

The Action of Ginseng

Ginseng, which means "man-shaped root," dates back to the first century B.C. Emperors enjoyed the medicinal use of ginseng and set aside special areas as imperial reserves for wild ginseng. Ginseng root, often resembling a human body, is good for all the organs in the body.

Ginseng research has been conducted in China, the Soviet Union, Britain, France, Italy, Japan, India, and the U.S.A. Ginseng's active substance contains glycosides, at least thirteen minerals and trace elements. The following therapeutic chemicals have been obtained from the ginseng root:

(1) *Panaxin and its related compounds* generally act as a stimulant for the midbrain, the heart, and the blood vessels.
(2) *Panax acid* acts as a stimulant for internal secretions.
(3) *Panaquilin* acts as a stimulant for internal secretions.
(4) *Panacen and Sapogenin,* both as volatile oils, can stimulate the central nervous system.
(5) *Ginseng* with the properties of lowering blood sugar.
(6) *Vitamins A, B1, B2, C, and possibly E.* (Some effects of ginseng are similar to those of Vitamin E).

Ginseng is, at least, a non-specific stimulant, if not a true panacea. It has anti-fatigue, anti-stress,, and anti-infective properties. Some researchers believe that it can delay the onset of the degenerative process of aging, thus prolonging life. It has hormonal effects and can strengthen sexual prowess. It is a tonic. The Russians have used ginseng to promote tissue growth and to increase mental and physical energy.

There are presently no known side effects from Panax Ginseng. However, if you are hyperactive, or pregnant or allergic to ginseng, do not take it.

Case Study

I saw a lady come into my clinic to buy three bottles of Panax Ginseng. Being curious, I asked her why she bought them. She responded that she had been in my workshop three weeks before, and it was the first time she had heard of ginseng for detoxifying the system and possibly relieving pain. She had pain in her elbow and had bought a bottle at the meeting. After two weeks, the pain disappeared with no other treatment, not even acupressure. She told me that she was buying three bottles for her son, who also had some pain problems.

I have not found any literature stating that ginseng can relieve pain. However, because of its detoxifying action, it restores the body to the normal functions of natural healing, which may indirectly release pain-supressing hormones.

CLINICAL APPLICATIONS OF SPECIFIC PAIN PROBLEMS

Alphabetical Order

All the pain problems are listed in alphabetical order. Under each pain problem are: (1) a brief description of the pain problem; and (2) the principle of treatment. Acupuncture/Acupressure points are arranged in the sequence in which they should be stimulated. Each point is named; its translation in parenthesis. It is followed by a description of the location, together with an illustration showing the relative anatomical position. That is followed by the stimulation technique, along with a picture showing live treatment. Remarks are added as necessary.

Very frequently, one problem has more than one symptom. In that case, you may start working on those points listed under that particular symptom and then on all points under that particular problem.

Body Posture

No matter what the subject's posture is — lying down, sitting up, or standing — your subject must be relaxed, comfortable, warm, and natural. There should be no crossed legs or tight clothing. The practitioner must be able to fully utilize finger movements and strength.

Cautions and Precautions

A. The practitioner
 1. Keep the treatment room warm but well ventilated. This will help the subject to be comfortable and prevent him from being chilled.
 2. The practitioner should keep his hands clean and warm, with his nails trimmed to prevent injuring the subject or making him tense and nervous. Nails should be shortened to extend just past the tip of the finger.
B. Patients and situations to avoid:
 1. Serious cardiac patients, especially those with pacemakers – it is very easy for these patients to pass out.
 2. Pregnant women. Some points, when stimulated, can cause miscarriage.
 3. Patients with contagious diseases.
 4. Nervous or terrified patients.

5. Tired, exhausted patients. Patients after strenuous exercise are also included.
6. Subjects with a full stomach. Working under this condition will not give the subject the full benefit of the treatment.
7. Subjects with an empty stomach. In this case the subject will be too weak to receive the stimulation.
8. Avoid working on skin surfaces with contusions, scars, or abrasions.
9. Never work on an eyeball, embolism, fracture, or open wound.
10. Stop treatments if symptoms are being aggravated and no relief is observed.

Finger Techniques

There are four ways of applying finger pressure: (1) finger nail, (2) finger tip, (3) finger ball, and (4) squeezing.

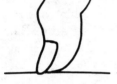

1. Finger nail pressure

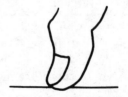

2. Finger tip pressure

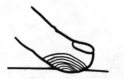

3. Finger ball pressure

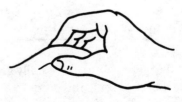

4. Squeezing

When applying pressure with the nail, tip, or ball of the finger, always keep your finger vertical to the designated point on the skin surface. Massage the point in static, small circular movements, about two or three cycles per second. Static movement means that your finger stays on the spot all the time. Do not scratch the skin surface or lift your finger. Otherwise, it is very easy to break the skin.

The pressure on each point should be about 10-15 pounds. This force of 10-15 pounds is a rather mechanical and ambiguous judgment. Proper judgment should be that you are generating some kind of sensation felt by the patient. This sensation can be felt as tenderness, soreness, numbness, or tingling. Many times, this sensation can travel up and down the area of the point being massaged. When this happens, it means that the patient is responding to the finger manipulation.

In other words, you don't just put your finger there and expect therapeutic results. You must be doing something. That something is generating the sensation.

At no time should the patient feel pain because of finger pressure. If this is the case, stimulate another point which is not painful. However, the patient should be able to clearly distinguish the difference between pain and sensation. Pain is not desirable; sensation is a good response and is more likely felt at spots where there are muscle bundles or nerve endings.

Most acupuncture points are located bilaterally. There will be better results if both points are stimulated simultaneously. This can be done with both hands once you have mastered the technique. Until then, you can start with one point at a time.

Frequency of Treatment

Finger pressure is usually given in periods ranging from a few seconds to one full minute for each point during which the subject feels the sensation.

Start counting after you have located the point, not while you are searching for it. You have to be generating the sensation.

You may apply stimulation once daily or whenever you have symptoms. I find that the best time to start treatment is when one feels on the verge of having symptoms. Some emergency points will require more than one minute.

The "Body Inch"

Since all of us are different in weight and height, we do not use the standard "inch" for locating the acupuncture/acupressure. The "body inch" is used. One body inch is defined as the distance between the two creases of the middle finger when the finger is bent. It is the patient's finger, not the practitioner's. Please note that throughout the series the term "inch" stands for "body inch."

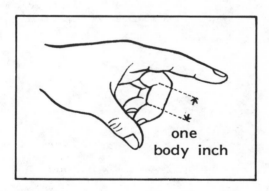

one
body inch

Important Note

You must study and thoroughly understand this entire chapter before attempting to work on any subject, including yourself. We recommend you read through it at least twice.

Let me emphasize that of all the modalities we have discussed in this book, no one modality is better than another. However, some patients do respond to one and not the other. Therefore, make sure all avenues are explored. For our purposes, I recommend the following: first try acupressure; then moxibustion (unless indicated as forbidden), and then auricular therapy. You may want to do body and auricular therapy at the same time. Meanwhile, all pain patients should follow the "forbidden diet." Panax Ginseng is highly recommended for pain patients, especially those who have taken pain medication and failed to respond. When in doubt, consult your acupuncturist or the author.

ABDOMINAL PAIN

At one time or another we all experience some stomach or abdominal pain. This is very common and, fortunately, can be easily controlled by acupressure or moxibustion.

Acute pain from acute or chronic gastritis, gastric and duodenal ulcers, spasms, enteritis, etc. can be relieved as indicated below. Acupressure is especially good for acute gastritis, which is usually caused by eating highly stimulating or contaminated food. Symptoms are sudden onset of nausea, vomiting, abdominal pain and diarrhea. These can be accompanied by headache, chills, and fever.

Pain from post-abdominal surgeries can also be relieved by acupressure, but avoid using points in the abdominal area.

Be aware that acute stomach pain is often a warning of serious illness which may require immediate surgical intervention. Conditions such as appendicitis, cholecystitis, acute peritonitis, perforated peptic ulcer, or cancer also cause pain in the abdominal area and do not indicate treatment by acupressure. Therefore, it is important that any chronic abdominal disorder be properly and thoroughly diagnosed before acupressure is tried.

Treatment

There are many points in both local and distal areas that are associated with the abdominal region. When these points are stimulated, they can generate peristalsis, which results in a rhythmic, wavelike motion of the walls of the alimentary canal. Very often, pain is reduced or relieved after the first treatment.

Note:
Other points are also chosen according to specific symptoms.
Moxibustion is also recommended.

SYMPTOM: Any Stomach or Abdominal Pain

Point: Stomach 36 *(Walk 3 miles)*

Location: About 3 inches below the knee cap, 1 inch lateral to the tibia.

Technique: Use the ball of the thumb to massage hard.

Remarks: Moxibustion is recommended.

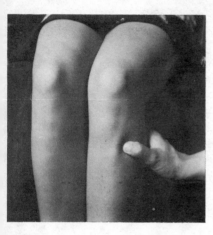
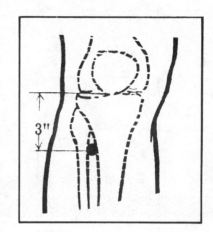

Point: Bladder 21 *(Stomach point)*

Location: About 1½ inches lateral to the lower border of the 12th thoracic vertebra.

Technique: Use the ball of the thumb to massage firmly. Ask the patient to lie down on the stomach.

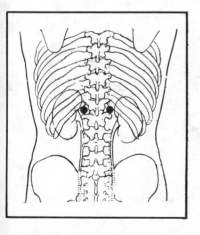
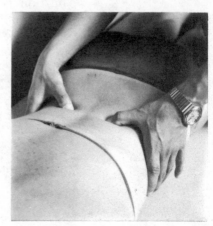

Point: Conception Vessel 12 *(Central Channel)*

Location: About 4 inches above the naval.

Technique: Press lightly over this point or use the squeezing technique.

Remarks: Moxibustion is recommended for stomach disorders. Avoid using this point for post-operative patients suffering from abdominal pain.

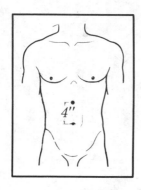 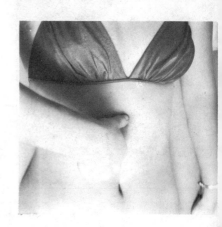

Point: O-yes Point *(Sensitive Point)*

Location: Anywhere surrounding the naval area.

Remarks: This is also known as the trigger point. Moxibustion is preferred over pressure. Avoid using this point for post-operative patients suffering from abdominal pain.

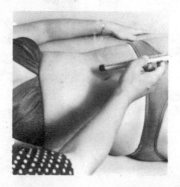

SYMPTOM: Nausea & Vomiting

Point: Pericardium 6 *(Inner Crate)*

Location: About 2 inches above the middle of the palmar wrist crease, in between the two tendons.

Technique: Use the fingernail to press down and massage.

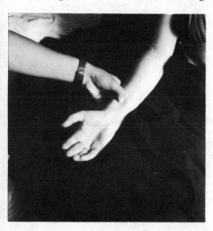
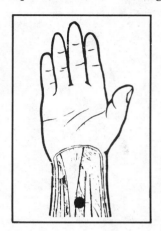

SYMPTOM: Food Poisoning

Point: Liver 3 *(Rush)*

Location: Between the 1st and 2nd toes, about 2 inches behind the margin of web.

Technique: Use fingernail to massage hard.

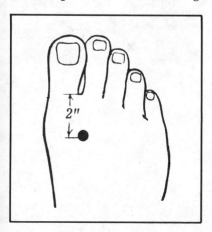
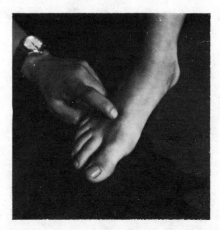

SYMPTOM: Dysentery

Point: Stomach 44 *(Inner Yard)*

Location: About ½ inch behind the web margin between the 2nd and 3rd toes.

Technique: Use fingernail to press hard.

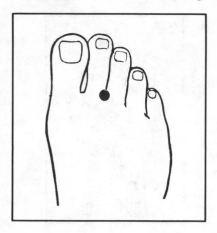

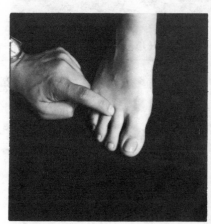

ALLERGIES

There are many types of allergies, but we shall limit o
discussion to only three; hayfever, rhinitis, and sinus. Becau
all of them have similar symptoms, the treatments will be mo
or less identical.

Acupressure may be used to reduce a person's general tenden
to react allergically as well as to treat the symptoms of allerg
Nasal congestion, discharge, itching, sneezing, swelling,
aching are usually relieved by acupressure.

Patients with allergic tendencies should avoid contact wi
known allergens.

It is recommended that treatment be used as a preventi
measure; use acupressure at the beginning of your aller;
season(s) each year.

Treatment

Points are chosen to relieve symptoms. "Stomach 36" enhanc
the therapeutic action of all points and reduces a person
general tendency to react allergically.

Note:
Moxibustion is also recommended on "Stomach 36."

SYMPTOM: see Allergies Symptoms including Headaches, Nasal Congestion, Discharge, Running Nose, etc.

Point: Governing Vessel 24.5 *(3rd Eye)*

Location: In between the eyebrows.

Technique: Use thumb and index fingers to squeeze and release several times.

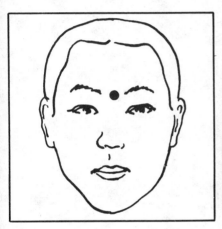 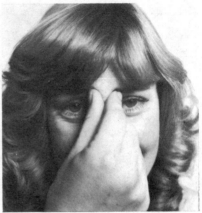

Point: Large Intestine 20 *(Welcome Fragrance)*

Location: By the side of the nose.

Technique: Use the index finger nail to massage.

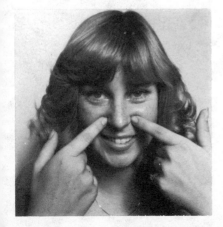 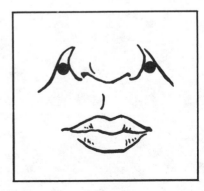

Point: Gall Bladder 20 *(Wind Pond)*

Location: At the depression below the occipital bone, about 1½ inches lateral to the midline of the head.

Technique: Use thumb tip to massage hard.

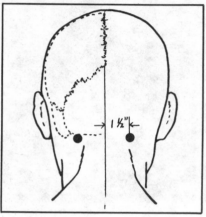

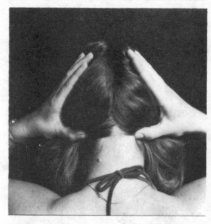

Point: Large Intestine 4 *(Meeting Valley)*

Location: At the highest spot of the muscle when the thumb and index finger are brought close together.

Technique: Use the thumb to press hard aiming at the point, but against the metacarpal bone of the index finger. Put one hand over the other to ensure the proper position and good grip.

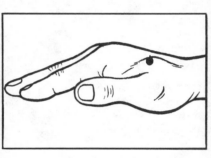 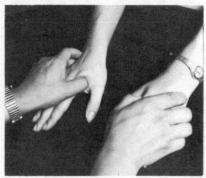

Point: Stomach 36 *(Walk 3 Miles)*

Location: 3 inches below the kneecap, 1 inch lateral to the tibia.

Technique: Use thumb ball to press hard.

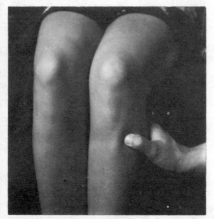 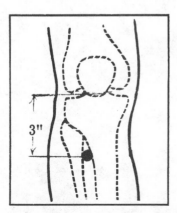

ARTHRITIS

Generally, arthritis can be classified into three types; rheumatic, rheumatoid, and osteoarthritis. All of them can be helped by acupressure, but it is not a cure. It can alleviate pain, lubricate the joints, ease inflammation and stiffness, and increase mobility. Healing will be difficult in the late stage if there is muscle atrophy, fusing of joints, deformity, inability to flex and extend the joint or permanent motor impairment. Therefore, it is suggested that you apply acupressure early when you begin to feel any symptoms such as aching, stiffness, or swelling of the joint(s).

Treatment

Points are chosen according to the disease-affected area(s).

To facilitate the process of healing, it is recommended that you move the affected area gently while treatment is being given.

Moxibustion is also indicated for arthritis and strongly recommended for all points. Do not apply moxibustion on an acutely inflamed area where there is local redness.

In order to consolidate the therapeutic effects and to restore functioning to the joints, some slow exercises are encouraged.

Point: Large Intestine 15 *(Shoulder Point)*

Location: At the depression of the acromion when the arm is raised.

Technique: Use the tip of the index finger to press hard.

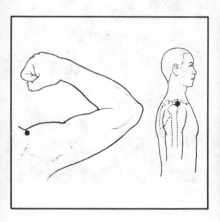
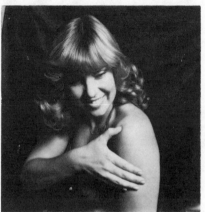

Point: Large Intestine 11 *(Crooked Pond)*

Location: At the external end of the elbow crease when the elbow is bent at a 90° angle.

Technique: Put the arm straight forward, then massage hard with the ball of the thumb.

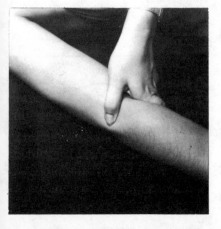
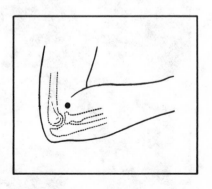

Point: Triple Warmer 5 *(Center Gate)*

Location: About 2 inches above the midpoint of the wrist crease, on the back of the wrist.

Technique: Use the tip of the finger to press hard.

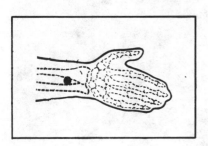

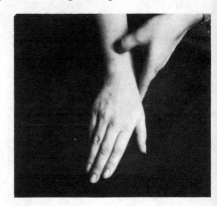

Point: Large Intestine 4 *(Meeting Valley)*

Location: At the highest spot of the muscle when the thumb and index finger are brought close together.

Technique: Use the thumb to press hard aiming at the point, but against the metacarpal bone of the index finger. Put one hand over the other to ensure the proper position and good grip.

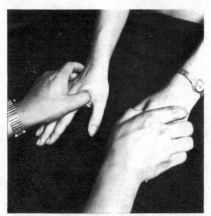

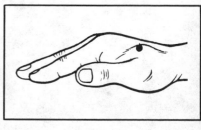

Point: Baxie *(8 Devils)*

Location: On the back of the hand, on the web between the 5 fingers of both hands, 8 points in all.

Technique: Use finger nail to massage.

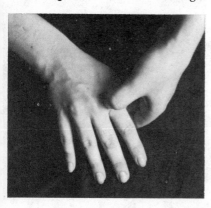 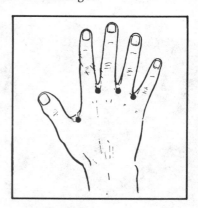

AFFECTED AREA: Lower Extremities

Point: Gall Bladder 30 *(Circle Jumping)*

Location: On the side of the buttock, at the junction of the hip joint.

Technique: Use thumb ball to press hard. Ask the subject to lie down in lateral recumbent position with thigh flexed.

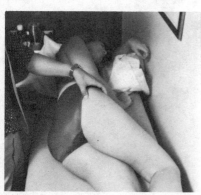 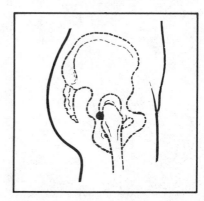

Point: Stomach 35 *(Tiger Eye)*

Location: In the depression just below the kneecap, on the external side.

Technique: Bend the knee at a 90° angle. Use the finger nail or tip to massage hard.

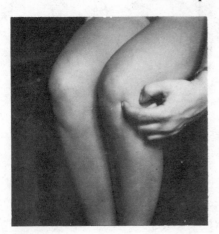 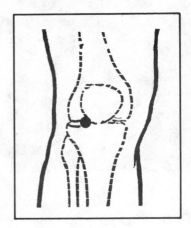

Point: Gall Bladder 34 *(Yang Spring Water)*

Location: In the depression 45° below the head of the fibula.

Technique: Use finger tip to press hard.

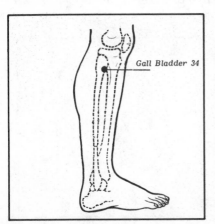 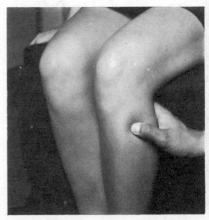

Point: Gall Bladder 39 *(Hanging Bell)*

Location: 3 inches above the external ankle, behind the fibula.

Technique: Use the thumb ball to press hard against the fibula.

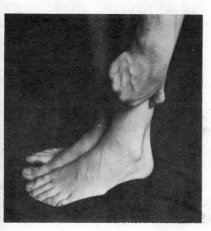 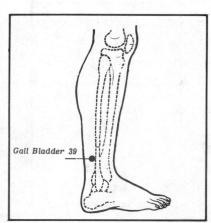

Point: Stomach 36 *(Walk 3 Miles)*

Location: 3 inches below the kneecap, 1 inch lateral to the tibia.

Technique: Use thumb ball to press hard.

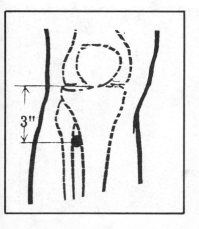 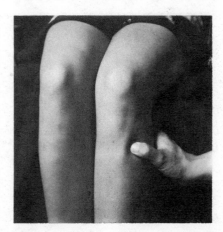

Point:	Stomach 41 *(Dissolving Stream)*
Location:	At the meeting of the top of foot and leg, in between the two tendons.
Technique:	Use finger nail to massage.

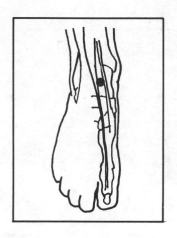 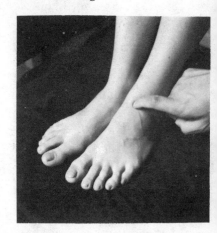

Point:	Gall Bladder 40 *(Soldem Mound)*
Location:	In the depression, at an angle of 45° below the external ankle.
Technique:	Use the finger nail to press down.

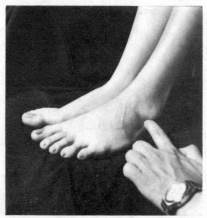 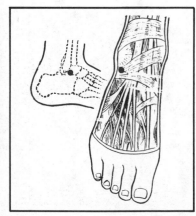

AFFECTED AREA: Lower Extremities (continued)

Point:	Bafeng *(8 Winds)*
Location:	On the back of foot, on the web between the 5 toes of both feet, 8 points in all.
Technique:	Use finger nail to massage.

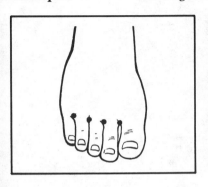

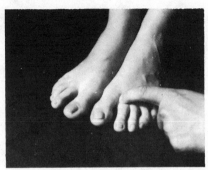

AFFECTED AREA: Vertebral Column

Point:	Huatuojiaji *(Two Sides of the Spine)*
Location:	On both sides of the spinal column, about ½ inch lateral to the midline. From the 1st cervical vertebra to the 4th sacral vertebra, there are 28 points altogether.
Technique:	Use finger tip or ball to massage corresponding points.

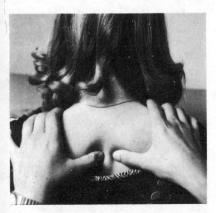

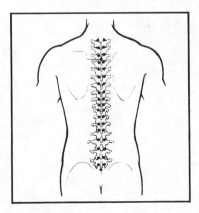

ELBOW AND ARM PAIN

There are three kinds of elbow pain frequently seen in the clinic: arthritis, tennis elbow, and acute lesion of the soft tissues of the elbow.

The main symptom is pain at the elbow. The pain may also be accompanied by swelling, stiffness, and impairment of movement of the involved limb. Sometimes, the pain spreads through the entire arm.

Should there be abnormal movement, bony crepitation, or fixed sensation, or should the deltoid configuration of the elbow be abnormal, seek medical attention to determine if a fracture or dislocation has occurred.

Acupressure is very effective in relieving elbow pain. It can make both subjective and objective symptoms fundamentally disappear and restore movement in the joint appreciably.

Treatment

Points are chosen according to the location of the pain. In addition to the points discussed here, the patient may also try some "O-yes" points (sensitive to pressure) at the painful area.

If there is no improvement or the point is too sore to press, massage the corresponding location on the healthy arm. Stretch and flex the limb when applying pressure to promote relaxation of the tendons and ligaments and to relieve the pain.

Note:
Moxibustion is also highly recommended.

SYMPTOM: Pain at the Elbow

Point: Large Intestine 11 *(Crooked Pond)*

Location: At the external end of the elbow crease when the elbow is bent at a 90° angle.

Technique: Put the arm straight forward, then massage hard with your thumb.

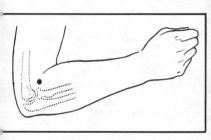

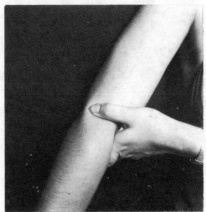

Point: Small Intestine 8 *(Small Sea)*

Location: At the internal end of the elbow crease when the elbow is bent at a 90° angle. Exactly opposite to Large Intestine 11.

Technique: Put the arm straight forward, then massage hard with your thumb.

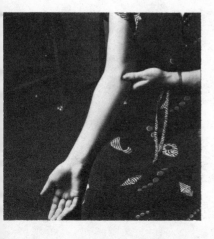

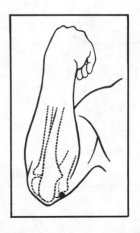

SYMPTOM: Pain in the Upper Arm or Shoulder

Point: Large Intestine 15 *(Shoulder Point)*

Location: At the depression of the acromion when the arm is raised.

Technique: Use the tip of the index finger to press hard.

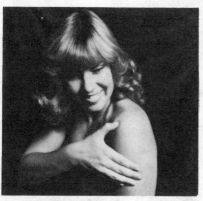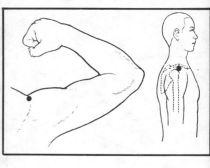

SYMPTOM: Pain in the Forearm

Point: Large Intestine 10 *(Hand 3 Miles)*

Location: About 2 inches directly below the external end of the elbow crease when the elbow is bent.

Technique: Use the ball of the thumb to press firmly.

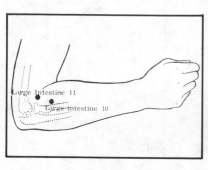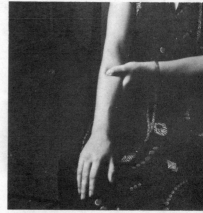

FACIAL, TRIGEMINAL
AND DENTAL PAIN

The facial area is served by the trigeminal nerve, which has three branches: the ophthalmic, the maxillary, and the mandibular. The ophthalmic branch is located over the upper third of the face, the maxillary over the middle third, and the mandibular over the lower third. Pain, such as trigeminal neuralgia, in any of these areas can be relieved by acupressure.

Dental pain is most commonly due to inflammation of the dental pulp, around the crown, periodontitis, dentoalveolar abscess, or dental caries. Acupressure is excellent in controlling such dental pain as TMJ pain dysfunction, toothache, and postoperative pain.

Treatment

Points are chosen according to innervation and channel of conduction to a specific area. Distal points are used in the upper and/or lower extremitites to ensure the local therapeutic actions.

Note:
Moxibustion is not used to alleviate facial, trigeminal or dental pain.

AFFECTED AREA: Upper Third of the Face

Point: Gall Bladder 14 *(Yang White)*

Location: About 1 inch above the midpoint of the eyebrow.

Technique: Use fingernail to press firmly.

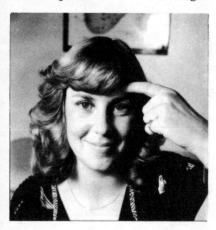 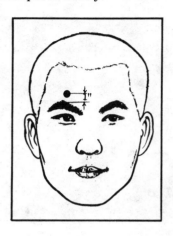

Point: Tai-yang *(The Sun)*

Location: Over the temple, in the depression about 1 inch behind the midpoint between the lateral end of the eyebrow and the outer corner.

Technique: Use the ball of the finger to massage lightly. Do not apply hard pressure.

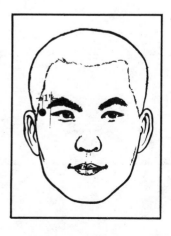 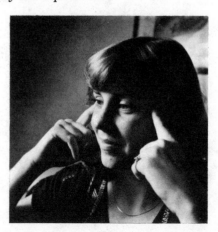

Point: Bladder 2 *(Drill Bamboo)*

Location: Over the inner end of the eyebrow, directly above the inner eye corner.

Technique: Use the tip of the finger to press hard.

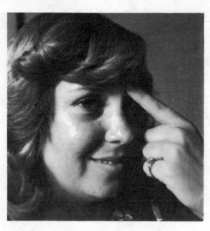
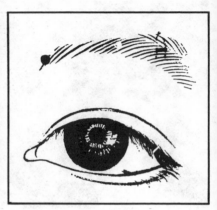

Point: Triple Warmer 5 *(Center Gate)*

Location: About 2 inches above the midpoint of the wrist crease, on the back of the wrist.

Technique: Use the tip of the finger to press hard.

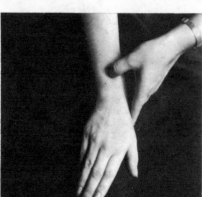
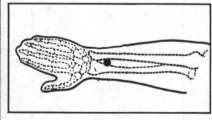

AFFECTED AREA: Middle Third of the Face

Point: Stomach 2 *(4 White)*

Location: At the lower end of the orbit, on the vertical level of the center of the pupil.

Technique: Use the tip of the finger to press hard.

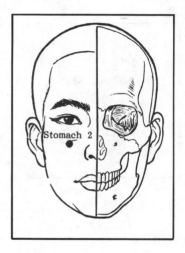 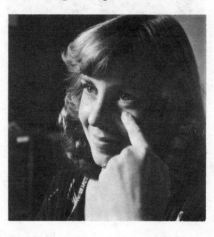

Point: Stomach 3 *(Big Bone)*

Location: On the same level with the nostril, directly on the vertical level of the center of the pupil.

Technique: Use the tip of the finger to press hard.

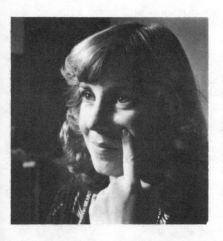 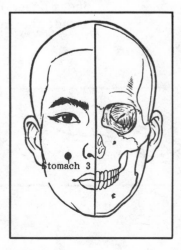

Point: Governing Vessel 26 *(The Center of the Man)*

Location: At the upper one-third of the philtrum.

Technique: Use the tip of the finger to press hard.

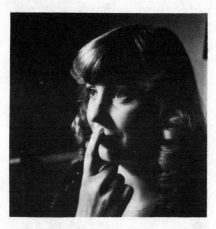

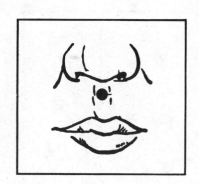

Point: Large Intestine 4 *(Meeting Valley)*

Location: At the highest spot of the muscle when the thumb and index finger are brought close together.

Technique: Use the thumb to press hard aiming at the point, but against the metacarpal bone of the index finger. Put one hand over the other to ensure the proper position and good grip.

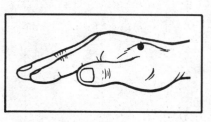

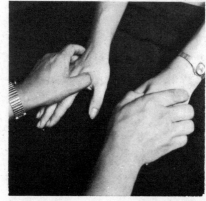

AFFECTED AREA: Lower Third of the Face

Point: Stomach 7 *(Lower Gate)*

Location: In the depression at the lower border of the zygomatic arch, about 1 inch in front of the tragus of the ear.

Technique: Use the tip of the finger to press hard.

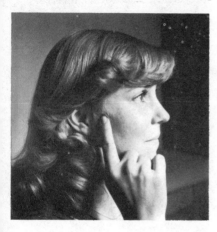 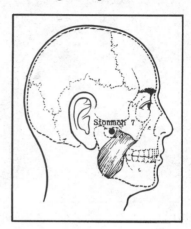

Point: Stomach 6 *(Cheek Chariot)*

Location: Directly over the prominence of the masseter muscle when the jaw is closed tight.

Technique: Use the ball of the finger to massage hard.

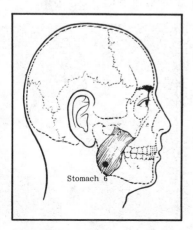 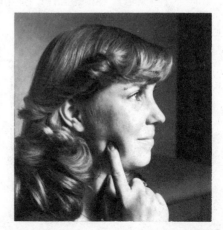

73

Point: Conception Vessel 24 *(Receiving Fluid)*

Location: On the midline and at the horizontal fold of the chin.

Technique: Use fingernail to press hard.

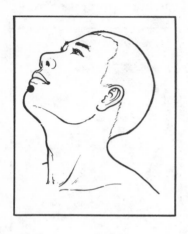 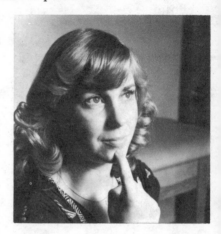

Point: Stomach 44 *(Inner Yard)*

Location: About ½ inch behind the web margin between the 2nd and 3rd toes.

Technique: Use fingernail to press hard.

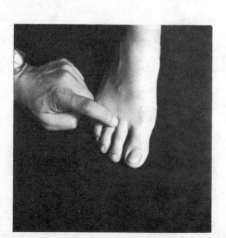 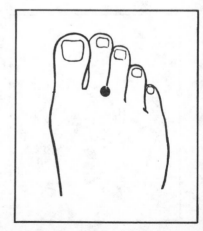

HEADACHES

The headache is merely a symptom of many conditions. Acupressure may help those conditions induced by: 1) diseases of the sense organs, e.g., sinusitis and glaucoma; 2) functional conditions, e.g., migraines, stress, tension or neurotic headaches; and 3) generalized diseases, e.g., hypertension, common cold, and influenza. Headaches caused by cerebral tumor, temporal arteries, focal inflammation, or meningitis will not be alleviated by acupressure.

After massage, the pressure or ache will be relieved. Usually after one or several treatments, the headache will be relieved or disappear.

Treatment

Points are chosen according to the origin of the headache. Whether it is a frontal, occipital, vertex, or migraine headache, "Large Intestine 4" is always used first to enhance the therapeutic action of any of those local points.

Note:
Moxibustion is not used here.

SYMPTOM: General Headache

Point: Large Intestine 4 *(Meeting Valley)*

Location: At the highest spot of the muscle when the thumb and index finger are brought close together.

Technique: Use the thumb to press hard aiming at the point, but against the metacarpal bone of the index finger. Put one hand over the other to ensure the proper position and good grip.

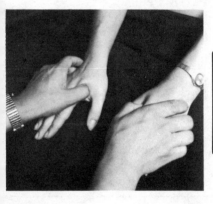 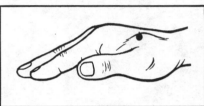

SYMPTOM: Pressure in Eyes

Point: Governing Vessel 24.5 *(3rd Eye)*

Location: In between the eyebrows.

Technique: Use thumb and index fingers to squeeze and release several times.

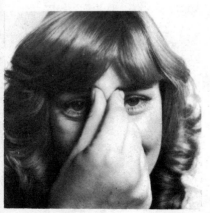 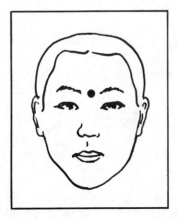

SYMPTOM: Tension at the Back of the Neck

Point:	Gall Bladder 20 *(Wind Pond)*
Location:	At the depression below the occipital bone, about 1½ inches lateral to the midline of the head.
Technique:	Use thumb tip to massage hard.

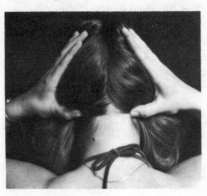 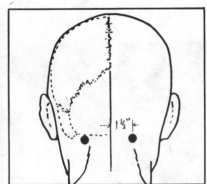

SYMPTOM: Migraines

Point:	Tai-yang *(The Sun)*
Location:	Over the temple, about 1 inch lateral to the midpoint between the end of the eyebrow and the outer canthus.
Technique:	Massage both points at the same time with your index finger balls. Do not apply hard pressure.

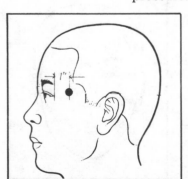 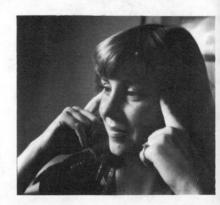

KNEE AND LEG PAIN

Knee pain is commonly caused by sprains. Since sprains cause lesions to soft tissues such as muscles, tendons, and ligaments, the pain may also be accompanied by swelling and impaired movement of the involved limb. There may be sharp pain when the knee joints are stretched or flexed to a certain position; the thigh may be weak and atrophic.

Pain caused by fracture, rupture, or dislocation of joints may not respond to acupressure. Even though acupressure may help temporarily, when the patient moves the limb, the pain may return.

Acupressure is, however, considered to be effective for border-line and small ruptures. Massage can make subjective and objective symptoms fundamentally disappear and restore the ability for physical activity. The success rate in this area is over 90%.

Treatment

Points are chosen according to the location of the pain. When massaging, put the knee at a 90 degree angle for better stimulation.

Note:
Moxibustion is also highly recommended.

SYMPTOM: Local Knee Pain

Point: Heding *(Crane Head)*

Location: On the midpoint of the upper boder of the knee cap.

Technique: Use the ball of the finger to massage hard.

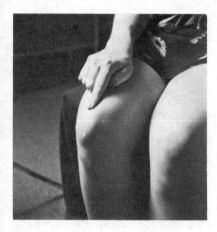
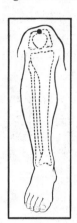

Point: Stomach 35 *(Tiger Eye)*

Location: In the depression just below the knee cap, on the external side.

Technique: Bend the knee at a 90° angle, use the finger nail or tip to massage hard.

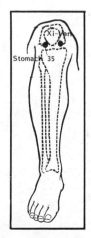
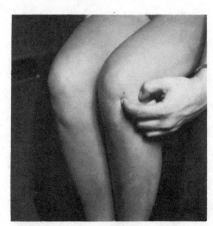

81

SYMPTOM: Local Knee Pain (continued)

Point: Xi-yan *(Tiger Eye)*

Location: In the depression just below the knee cap, on the internal side.

Technique: Bend the knee at a 90° angle, use the finger nail or tip to massage hard.

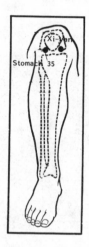

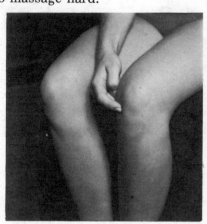

SYMPTOM: Pain Spreading to the Leg

Point: Gall Bladder 34 *(Yang Spring Water)*

Location: In the depression at an angle of 45° below the head of the fibula.

Technique: Use the tip of the finger to press hard.

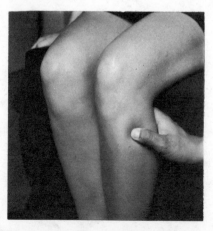

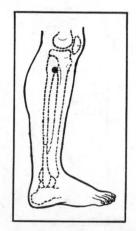

SYMPTOM: Pain Spreading to the Leg (continued)

Point: Stomach 36 *(Walk 3 Miles)*

Location: About 3 inches below the knee cap, 1 inch lateral to the tibia.

Technique: Use the ball of the thumb to press hard.

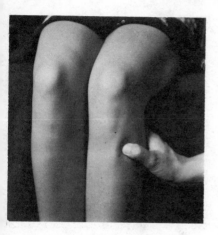
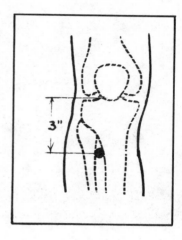

LEG AND ANKLE PAIN

Leg and ankle pain are commonly caused by arthritis or sprains. Sprains, which cause lesions in soft tissues, muscles, tendons, and ligaments, are generally due to sudden movements such as falls or unexpected pressure. Sprains primarily occur at the joint and elicit local pain, swelling, and impaired movement of the involved limb. Sprains do not include fractured bones or dislocated joints.

Acupressure is also considered very effective for borderline and small ruptures. Massage can make subjective and objective symptoms fundamentally disappear and restore the ability for physical activity.

Treatment

Points are chosen according to the location of the pain.

If there is no result or the point is too sore to apply pressure, massage the corresponding location on the healthy side. Stretch and flex the limb while applying pressure to promote relaxation of the tendons and ligaments and to relieve the pain.

Note:
Moxibustion is also highly recommended.

Point: Gall Bladder 34 *(Yang Spring Water)*

Location: In the depression 45° below the head of the fibula.

Technique: Use finger tip to press hard.

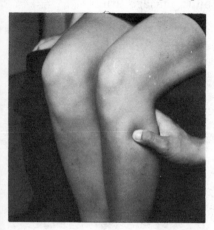

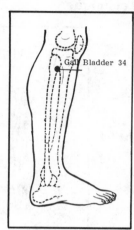

Point: Gall Bladder 39 *(Hanging Bell)*

Location: About 3 inches above the tip of the external ankle, behind the fibula.

Technique: Use the thumb to press hard against the fibula.

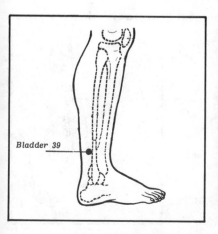

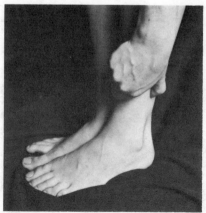

Point: Stomach 41 *(Dissolving Stream)*

Location: At the meeting of the top of foot and leg, between the two tendons.

Technique: Use fingernail to masage firmly.

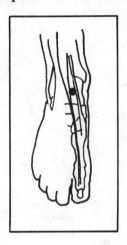
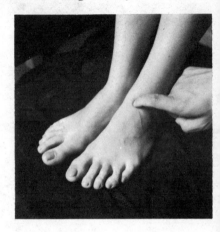

Point: Gall Bladder 40 *(Soldem Stream)*

Location: In the depression, at an angle of 45° below the external ankle.

Technique: Use the fingernail to press down.

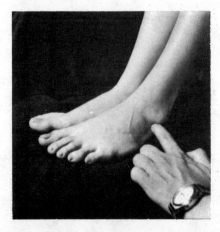
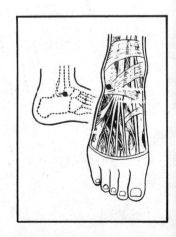

Point: Bladder 60 *(The Mountain)*

Location: Behind the external ankle, on the same level with the tip of the ankle.

Technique: Use the fingernail to press hard.

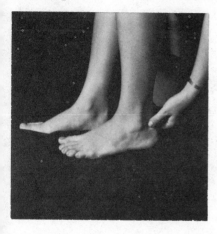

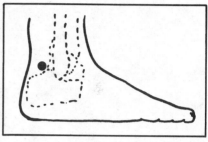

LOWER BACK PAIN

Lower back pain is a very common symptom caused by various etiological factors: sprain, strain, arthritis, slipped disc, pinched nerve, etc. Often the pain radiates from the lower back down to the back of the thigh and leg. This is called sciatica. Fortunately, acupressure has proven to be very effective in treating the above conditions.

Patients with a history of surgery(ies), such as laminectomy, will have a poor response to acupressure in this area.

Treatment

Points are chosen according to the location of the pain. Even though you are experiencing positive results, avoid aggravating the condition by staying away from strenuous exercises or hard work involving heavy physical activities.

Note:
Moxibustion is also recommended.

SYMPTOM: Local Lower Back Pain

Point: Governing Vessel 4 *(Life Door)*

Location: Located between the 2nd and 3rd lumbar vertebra, on the same level with the naval.

Technique: Use thumb tip to massage. Ask patient to lie down on the stomach.

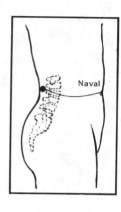

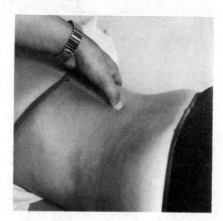

Point: Bladder 23 *(Kidney Point)*

Location: About 1½ inches lateral to the lower end of the 2nd lumbar vertebra, on the same level with the naval.

Technique: Use thumb ball to press hard toward the spine. Ask patient to lie down on the stomach.

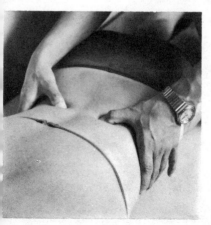

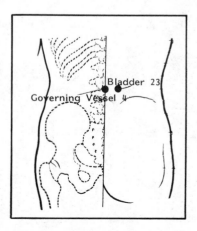

SYMPTOM: Pain at Lower Back or/and Leg

Point: Bladder 54 *(Commanding Center)*

Location: Exact midpoint of the crease of the knee back.

Technique: Use thumb and index fingers to squeeze or finger tip to press.

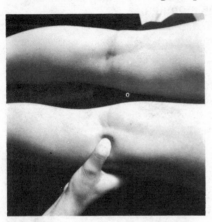 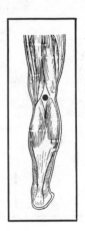

SYMPTOM: Pain Behind or Around the Leg

Point: Gall Bladder 34 *(Yang Spring Water)*

Location: In the depression 45° below the head of the fibula.

Technique: Use finger tip to press hard.

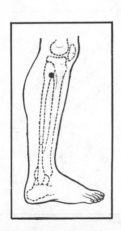 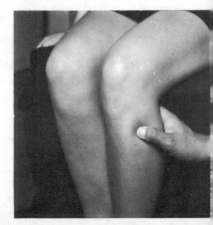

MENSTRUAL PAIN
AND DISCOMFORT

Menstrual disorders include scanty menses, painful menses, irregular menstrual cycle, pre-menstrual tension, excessive menstruation, prolonged or shortened menses, too dark or too light blood, etc. These menstrual dysfunctions may be due to dysfunction of the ovary and disturbance of the menstrual cycle.

Lack of menses may be due to disorder of endocrine function or generalized chronic disease, such as pulmonary tuberculosis, anemia, malnutrition, hypoplasia of uterus, turberculosis, of the genital organs, etc.

It is important to note that any menstrual disorder, especially excessive menstruation, requires prompt medical attention. Standard medical treatment should be used before acupressure.

Acupressure is effective in relieving pre-menstrual pain and regulating the menstrual cycle.

Treatment

There are points known as "female points." "Spleen 6," in Chinese called "three females meeting together," (so named because all three meridians on the leg meet at the point) is an excellent point for treating menstrual disorders.

Note:
Moxibustion is also recommended.
If pain is involved, watch your diet. (See chapter on Diet Therapy.)

SYMPTON: Pain or Discomfort in Abdominal Area

Point: Spleen 6 *(Female Point)*

Location: About 3 inches above the tip of the internal ankle, behind the tibia.

Technique: Use the ball of the thumb to massage hard.

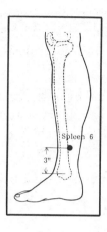

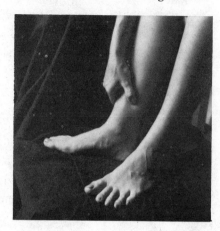

Point: Spleen 9 *(Yin Spring Water)*

Location: In the depression on the lower border of the end of the tibia, on the medial side.

Technique: Use the tip of the finger to massage hard.

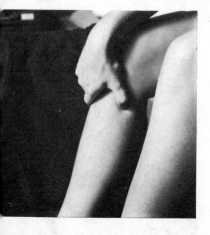

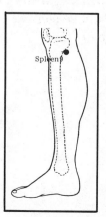

Point:	Spleen 10 *(Blood Sea)*
Location:	About 2 inches above the upper border of the knee cap, at the middle of the bulge of the muscle.
Technigue:	Use the ball of the thumb to massage firmly.

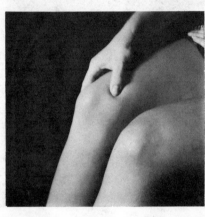 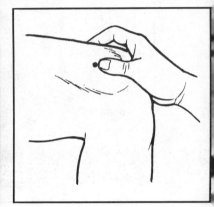

Point:	Conception Vessel 4 *(Gate Source)*
Location:	About 3 inches below the naval.
Technique:	Use the ball of the finger to massage firmly or use the squeezing technique. Do not press down to hard, because there is no hard structure below this point and you may hurt the internal organs.

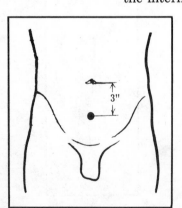 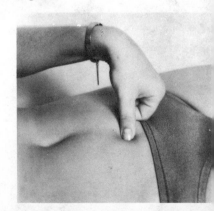

SYMPTOM:Pain and Discomfort in Abdominal Area (cont'd.)

Point: Bladder 23 *(Kidney Point)*

Location: About 1½ inches lateral to the lower end of the 2nd lumbar vertebra, on the same level with the naval.

Technique: Use the ball of the thumb to press hard toward the spine. Ask patient to lie down on the stomach.

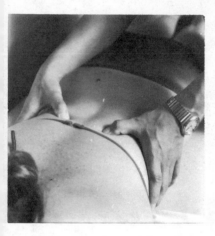
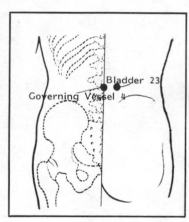

NECK PAIN AND
WHIPLASH INJURIES

Pain, stiffness, and muscular spasms of the neck are often caused by arthritis and cervical disc pathology. Whiplash injuries, usually caused by automobile accidents, result from sudden overextension of the neck.

Neck pain is very common. The neck carries the considerable weight of the head; it is fragile and easily hurt. Pressure and tension constantly build up in the neck muscle and cause pain.

Sometimes, as a result of neck injury, aches and/or numbness may occur in the hands and fingers. This condition may be due to a pinched spinal nerve in the neck.

Treatment

Points are chosen according to symptoms. Move your head from side to side and up and down when massaging the distal points. This will facilitate healing.

Note:
Moxibustion is recommended for the shoulder; it is not used on the neck and head.

SYMPTOM: Stiffness and Pain in the Neck

Point: Gall Bladder 20 *(Wind Pond)*

Location: At the depression below the occipital bone, about 1½ inches lateral to the midline of the head.

Technique: Use the tip of your thumb to massage hard. Bend your head forward.

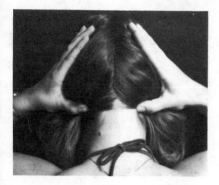
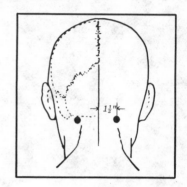

Point: Governing Vessel 14 *(Big Hammer)*

Location: In between the 7th cervical and the 1st thoracic vertebrae.

Technique: Use fingernail to massage. Make sure the fingernail is perpendicular and that the pressure applied is between the two discs. Bend the head forward when massaging.

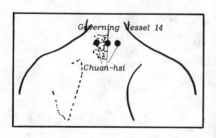
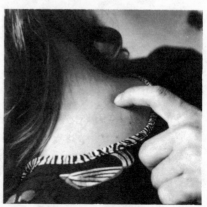

103

Point: Chuan-hsi *(Panting Point)*

Location: Immediately lateral to the lower end of the 7th cervical disc.

Technique: Use the tip of the finger to massage firmly. Bend the head forward when massaging.

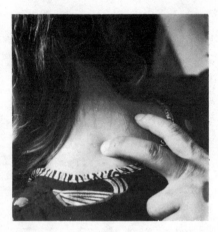

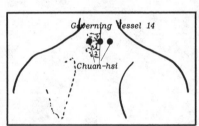

Point: Small Intestine 3 *(Back Stream)*

Location: Located at the end of the transverse crease, on the border of the palm below the little finger.

Technique: Use fingernail to press hard.

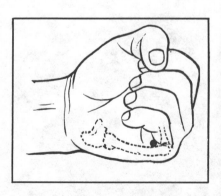

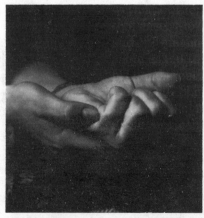

SHOULDER PAIN

A painful shoulder often occurs as a symptom due to sprain or strain of the soft tissues surrounding the shoulder joint. This may cause: 1) perifocal inflammation of the shoulder joint; 2) supraspinatus tendinitis; 3) infra-acromial bursitis; and 4) tendosynovitis of the long head of biceps brachaii.

All of these cause pain, limited movement, swelling, tenderness, or stiffness when raising or stretching the arm. The pain may cover a large area and radiate to the arm and elbow.

Acupressure can relieve all of the above symptoms. The rate of success is over 90%. Acupressure is likely to fail if there is calcium deposit around the shoulder joint or if there is muscular atrophy.

Treatment

Both local and distal points are chosen. Symptomatic relief may be seen immediately after the first treatment.

Move your shoulder joint when stimulating distal points. This will assist in eliminating aches and stiffness.

Note:
Moxibustion is highly recommended and should be tried for better relief.

Point:	Large Intestine 15 *(Shoulder Point)*
Location:	At the depression of the acromion when the arm is raised.
Technique:	Use the tip of the index finger to press hard.

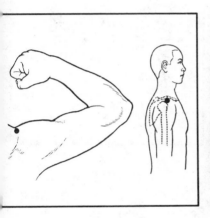 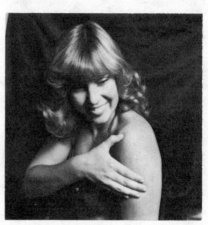

Point:	Chien-chien *(Shoulder Spot)*
Location:	About 1 inch above the anterior axillary fold.
Technique:	Use the tip of the finger to press hard.

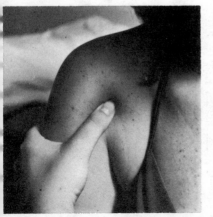 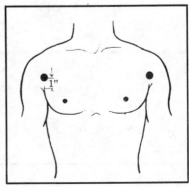

SYMPTOM: Pain across the Shoulder

Point: Gall Bladder 21 *(Shoulder Well)*

Location: On the hump of the shoulder.

Technique: Use the ball of the finger to press firmly or use the squeezing technique to pinch the point.

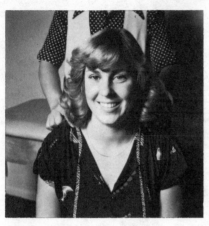
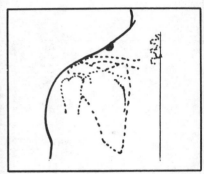

Point: Large Intestine 11 *(Crocked Pond)*

Location: At the external end of the elbow crease when the elbow is bent at a 90° angle.

Technique: Put the arm straight forward, then massage hard with the ball of the thumb.

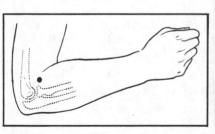
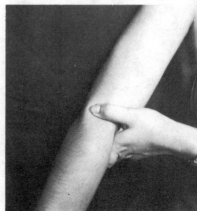

Point: Gall Bladder 34 *(Yang Spring Water)*

Location: In the depression 45° angle below the head of the fibula.

Technique: Use the tip of the finger to press hard.

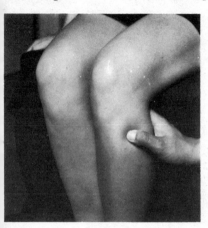
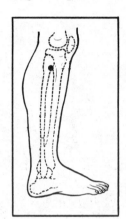

Point: Stomach 36 *(Walk 3 Miles)*

Location: About 3 inches below the knee cap, 1 inch lateral to the tibia.

Technique: Use the ball of the thumb to press hard.

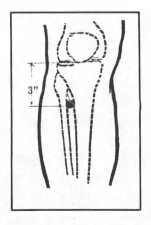
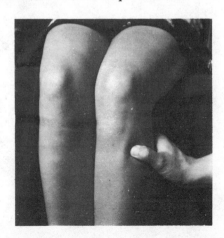

WRIST, HAND AND FINGER PAIN

Wrist, hand, and finger pains are commonly caused by arthritis or muscular-skeletal disorders, which cause lesions in soft tissues such as muscles, tendons, and ligaments. In instances of bone fracture or joint dislocation, seek medical attention.

The main symptom is pain at the local area. Pain may also be accompanied by swelling, stiffness, numbness, and impairment of movement of the involved wrist, hand, and/or fingers.

Acupressure is considered to be very effective for pain in these regions. It can make subjective and objective symptoms fundamentally disappear and restore the ability to engage in physical activity.

Treatment

Points are chosen according to the location of the pain. In addition, "O-yes" points (sensitive to pressure) in the painful area may be tried.

If there is stiffness and pain in the finger joints, massage both sides of the knuckles on the back of the hand.

Stretch and flex the afflicted wrist, hand, or finger while applying pressure to promote relaxation of the tendons and ligaments of the sprained location and relieve the pain.

Note:
Moxibustion is also highly recommended.

SYMPTOM: Pain in the Wrist

Point:	Small Intestine 6 *(Keep the Old)*
Location:	Flex elbow with palm placed on the chest; the point is on the bony cleft on the radial aspect of the ulna head.
Technique:	Use the fingernail to press firmly.

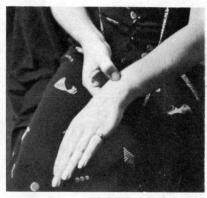
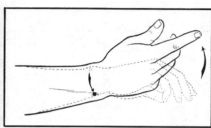

SYMPTOM: Pain at the Thumb

Point:	Large Intestine 5 *(Yang Stream)*
Location:	On the radial side of the back of the wrist. When the thumb is tilted upward, it is in the hollow between the two tendons.
Technique:	Use the fingernail to massage firmly.

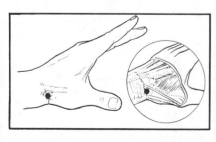
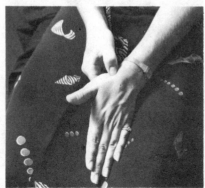

SYMPTOM: Pain at the Thumb (continued)

Point: Lung 7 *(Listing Deficiency)*

Location: When the index fingers and thumbs of both hands are crossed, the point is in the depression right under the tip of the index finger. Above the radius head.

Technique: Use the fingernail to massage firmly.

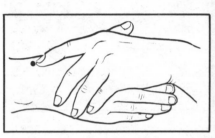 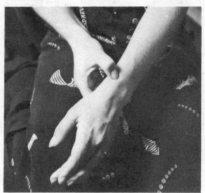

SYMPTOM: Pain at the Index and/or Middle Fingers

Point: Pericardium 7 *(Big Mound)*

Location: At the midpoint of the transverse crease of the wrist between the two tendons.

Technique: Use the fingernail to massage firmly.

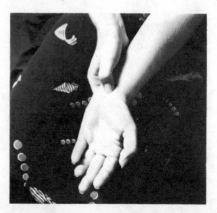 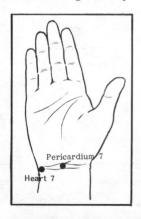

114

SYMPTOM: Pain at the Little Finger

Point: Heart 7 *(Divine Gate)*

Location: At the depression below the crease of the wrist, on the side of the little finger.

Technique: Bend your wrist, then use fingernail to massage firmly.

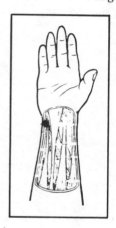
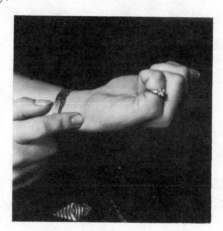

SYMPTOM: Numbness and/or Pain in the Hand

Point: Lung 10 *(Fish Side)*

Location: On the palmar surface, in the middle of the 1st metacarpal bone.

Technique: Use the tip of the finger to press hard.

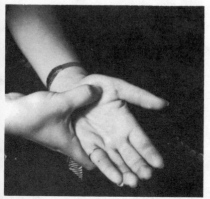
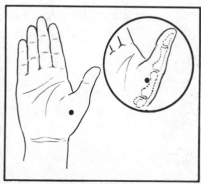

CASE STUDIES AND OTHER COMMENTS

NAME: P.O.   AGE: 39   SEX: Female

Present Complaints: Headaches – usually on the right side over and behind the eyes; sometimes a band of pressure around the head; other times just at sinus points, back of head and neck only.

Diagnosis by Patient's Doctor: Migraine aggravated by allergy-sinus.

Cause of Pain: Allergy – change of weather; menstruation; tension.

Length of Pain: Approximately 25 years.

Degree of Pain: From moderate to unbearable. Usually severe.

Medication: Analgesics including narcotics.

Previous or Present Treatments: Moist heat, dry heat, dark room treatment (when severe), no movement or talking.

Treatment and Result: The patient had severe headaches when acupressure was performed on her. Two "Large Intestine 4" points were massaged at the same time. The patient claimed immediate relief; however, there was still some pressure over the eyes and the temple. Two "Tai-yang" and "Governing Vessel 24.5" were then stimulated. The patient claimed 90% of the pain disappeared. When contacted about three months later, she reported that the headaches were getting much better with acupressure self-treatment. Even though her head hurt sometimes, it was bearable. However, she said she did not do well when she went to Minnesota for three-weeks vacation. During her stay there, the weather was warm and humid, which might have caused her problem. Also, she had hurt her leg and was taking medication for it. This might have been the factor in blocking the stimulation. As I talked to her, she said she was glad to be back in California because the headaches no longer bothered her as much.

CASE STUDY: Headaches

NAME: M.R.   **AGE: 31**   **SEX: Female**

Present Complaints: Frontal Headache.
Cause of Pain: Tension from hangover the previous night.
Length of Pain: Four hours.
Treatment and Result: The patient's headache was described as moderate when acupressure was performed. No medication was taken by the patient. After massaging two "Large Intestine 4" point, the headache was completely gone according to the patient. She was contacted the next day and was still well.

NAME: I.G.   AGE: 70   SEX: Female

Present Complaints: Lower back pain with muscular cramps.
Diagnosis by Patient's Doctor: Slipped disc at first lumbar.
Cause of Pain: From lift.
Length of Pain: Ten years, on and off.
Degree of Pain: From severe to unbearable at the time of treatment.
Medication: Darvon.
Previous or Present Treatment: Physiotherapy, chiropractics, wearing of a brace.
Treatment and Result: "Gall Bladder 34" and "Stomach 36" were massaged on both legs. According to the patient, 70% of the pain was relieved after the stimulation. The patient was contacted two-and-a-half months later and claimed to be greatly improved. No point had been stimulated since, but ginseng had been taken.

NAME: P.L.   AGE: 33   SEX: Male

Present Complaints: Lower back pain and right arch pain.
Cause of Pain: Accident.
Length of Pain: Three years.
Degree of Pain: Severe.
Medication: None.
Treatment and Result: At the time of the treatment, the patient was instructed to bend his back and try to reach the floor with his hands. He did it with great pain, and his hands were about ten inches from the floor. Moxibustion was used in this case. Moxa therapy was used on both "Gall Bladder 34" and "Stomach 36" and then on "Spleen 6". The patient was again asked to bend his back. He did it with no pain, and both his hands reached the floor with ease. He claimed there was no pain at all. The patient was contacted one week later and said he had been playing soccer all week long with no pain. He had been using moxa therapy and taking ginseng.

CASE STUDY: Shoulder Pain

NAME: E.M.   AGE: 67   SEX: Female

Present Complaints: Severe pain at the right shoulder, radiating up the back of the head and down the arm to the wrist and into the knuckle of the thumb.

Cause of Pain: Unknown

Length of Pain: About 35 years, on and off; severe to unbearable for the last three weeks.

Medication: None.

Previous or Present Treatment: None.

Treatment and Result: Two "Large Intestine 15" were stimulated one by one. The patient claimed better movement and 90% relief of the pain. The patient was contacted about 75 days later and claimed that the improvement had been maintained. The pain had become bearable. She said she was not taking any ginseng, but she felt she should.

NAME: H.R.   AGE: 64   SEX: FEMALE

Present Complaints: Restricted motion of the right arm – pain in the shoulder. Restriction of motion has increased in the past two years.

Diagnosis: ?

Cause of Pain: Auto accident 15 years ago – struck her shoulder on the dashboard.

Length of Pain: Intermittent pain for 14-15 years.

Degree of Pain: Varying from mild to moderate.

Medication: None.

Treatment and Result: "Large Intestine 15" was stimulated on the afflicted shoulder point. The patient immediately claimed relief from the pain and better movement of her shoulder. She was contacted about three months later and said there had been no recurrence of the shoulder pain and mobility problem. She was satisfied with one demonstration on just one point.

CASE STUDY: Temporal Mandibular Joint Pain and Myofacial Syndrome

NAME: S.D.   AGE: 43   SEX: Female

Present Complaints: Facial pain – could barely open mouth.
Diagnosis by Patient's Doctor: TMJ and myofacial syndrome.
Cause of Pain: By accident and possible stress.
Length of Pain: Several years and getting worse with age.
Degree of Pain: Unbearable at the time of treatment.
Medication: Asprin and norpramin.
Previous or Present Treatment: Acupuncture, physical therapy, ultrasound, chiropractics, and presently a dentist's care.
Treatment and Result: At the time of the demonstration, the patient could barely open her mouth, and only then with great pain. Local points "Stomach 6 and 7" were first tried, which seemed to aggravate her problem. Distal points were then chosen. Two "Large Intestine 4" were massaged. The patient responded with about 50% ease of pain and could open her mouth halfway. Two "Gall Bladder 34" were then stimulated. The patient claimed immediate and complete relief from the pain. Also, she could open her mouth all the way without pain. The treatment was performed around 10 a.m. and by 5 p.m the same day, the relief was still present. The patient was contacted about ten days later regarding her problem and said the relief lasted for only two days. Since then she had not done any acupressure on herself. When I asked her why, she told me she was under her dentist's care and would like to give him a chance before using any other method. I then told her to get in touch with me if she was still in pain when finished with the dentist's treatment. I felt that since she responded so well to the first treatment, she would continue to do so if she would follow the instruction properly.

This reminds me of another case in one of my workshops. I was demonstrating on a participant who could barely open her mouth. It was so tightly closed, she could barely eat or talk. This condition had been with her for at least seven years. I worked on the local points, "Stomach 6 and 7". Immediately, she was able to open her mouth halfway. The next morning, I did it one more time; she was able to open her mouth at will for the first time in seven years.

What Workshop Participants Say

In the past few years, I have been setting up one or two day acupressure workshops in major cities across the country. More than 5,000 health care professionals have received my personal training. Following is a list of sample comments from previous participants:

". . . Opened new vistas regarding pain and the relieving of pain without using drugs . . . intriguing subject matter – subject of arthritis and relating diet." – A.G. of McAllen, TX.

"Everything is just excellent." – N.M. of Chicago, IL.

"I thoroughly enjoyed the classes and certainly believe that acupressure could become an important part of 'Western Medicine'. I have used acupressure on some of my friends since the class with good results. I am looking forward to your next acupressure workshop." – G.G. of Palatka, FL.

"Over the years I've attended many classes, seminars, etc. as both a nurse and a physician's wife. Never has one been so full of information and so well presented as yours here this last week. You truly have a gift of being informative and making the class fun. We all came away feeling you had become our friend." – B.G. of Sacramento, CA.

"Integrated all facets of Chinese medicine." – B.J. of Park City, NJ.

"Your presentation of areas we can all utilize in many ways to make our health even better was super. Not a dull moment, and the actual workshop experience has helped Fern and me to put them to use already. We feel with further study and practice we will be prepared for a healthy and happy future, knowing we can maintain our health, drive, and energy longer than would have been thought possible." – R.G. of Van Nuys, CA.

"I attended your acupressure workshop at the Chicago Marriott. I am thrilled with my new skill to assist people with their pain, especially headaches. My co-workers are astonished at the fast results and the ability to help themselves." – C.B. of Skokie, IL.

What Experts Say About Dr. Chan

"I just finished reviewing your book and I want to make a few comments about it because I think it's a very important contribution to the literature of acupuncture and acupressure. Since 1972 when acupuncture first really came on the scene in the United States, I have been aware that you were a major pioneer in the field. You were holding forth educational material for doctors when they were seeking it and trying to understand what acupuncture was, and you have been consistent in continuing that through the intervening years. In your book, your pictures are accurate and understandable and make it possible for anyone, with a moderate degree of effort, to learn how to use acupressure for a variety of problems of the human body. So it is with a great deal of pleasure that I highly recommend your book to anyone who wants to learn acupressure."

William M. McGarey, M.D.
A.R.E. Clinic, Phoenix, AZ.

"Dr. Chan's procedures and choice of points are examples of his tremendous knowledge and the amount of research he has done in the field of acupressure."

Paul Hoffmeister, D.O., O.M.D.
Director, American Institute of
Chinese Medicine
Wailuku, Maui, HI.

"From over 25 years experience in the field, I can say that of all the books written in recent years about acupuncture/acupressure, Dr. Chan's are by far the most usable for practical application by the layman and professional alike."

K.E. Schulz, M.D. (Hom), D.C.,
Certified Acupuncturist
Holistic Bio-Medical Clinic,
San Luis Obispo, CA.

WHY SOME PEOPLE DO NOT RESPOND TO TREATMENT AND WHAT TO DO ABOUT IT

Introduction

It is very important to look upon pain sufferers as whole beings. When you examine pain victims, make sure they are completely relaxed, comfortable, and free from distractions, both inside and outside the body. When you help them achieve this optimal condition, your rate of success in controlling pain should be 90% or greater. In the course of my experiences in dealing with my pain patients, I have literally found it true that an ounce of prevention is worth a pound of cure. It is imperative to weigh the benefits and detriments of surgery and drug therapy vs. acupuncture/acupressure therapy.

Surgery

This refers to patients who have had surgery, one or more times, for the same pain problem(s) for which they now seek acupuncture /acupressure therapy. Due to surgical intervention, the patient's system may be in a state of confusion or stimulation channels may be interrupted. Most patients who fail to respond to acupuncture/acupressure fall into this category. This does not mean that patients who still suffer from pain after surgery cannot benefit from acupuncture/acupressure. Chances for successfully controlling pain in post-surgery pain patients are entirely dependent on the individual problem(s).

My suggestion is: prevention is far better than cure. When you are considering surgery for your pain problem, get an opinion from an acupuncturist or physician trained in acupuncture, or simply try acupuncture three or four times. If it does not work, you can always seek surgery. If it helps, and most of the time it will help, it will save you time, money, possible complications and side effects, tissue damage, and unnecessary suffering.

Don't misunderstand that you should try acupuncture/acupressure for everything before undergoing surgery. Acupuncture also has limits. Certainly, if you have appendicitis and surgery is indicated, submit to surgery. If you have a fractured shoulder, hip, or knee, see an orthopedic surgeon. Try acupuncture when no known cause is found for your pain, or even when the cause is known, but the rate of cure is low (e.g., lower back pain, sciatica, bursitis, persistent headaches), or when surgery poses a great risk.

Drugs

When patients have been taking drugs for two or more weeks and seek acupuncture/acupressure treatment, they may not respond optimally to the stimulation. Drug action may block the effects of acupuncture/acupressure stimulation. In traditional Chinese medicine, this may mean that the internal energy is not properly conducted in the stimulation channels.

Dr. Richard Kroening, Director of the UCLA Pain Management Clinic, claims that drugs often supress the functions of the pituitary glands, thus inhibiting them from releasing hormones which may induce pain relief.

Acupuncture/acupressure works on one's own natural healing system. If drugs turn off this system, acupuncture/acupressure may not work for a time. However, when the effects of the drugs wear off, acupuncture/acupressure often works. When we talk about drugs, I refer mostly to the following: pain killers, such as asprin, darvon, tylenol and their compounds; narcotic agents, such as codeine, demerol, and morphine; anti-inflammatory agents, such as cortisone; anti-depressants, such as tofranil and elavil; and tranquilizers, such as valium and librium. If you have been on any of the above drugs, I would suggest you consult the physician who prescribed the drug and ask if you could stop taking it before seeking acupuncture/acupressure therapy.

Please take note that if you have been taking a drug for some time and suddenly stop, you may develop withdrawal symptoms which may make you nervous and irritable.

While you are off drugs, I would recommend you take Panax Ginseng to help restore your normal natural healing powers. (Please refer to the chapter on Herbal Therapy Using Ginseng.) If you are responding to drug therapy and getting satisfactory relief, by all means continue taking the drug. However, if you are not gaining the response you expect, stop taking the drug and seek other help.

From the Author

Many of my professional colleagues, workshop participants, patients and friends have benefitted from my work in acupuncture/acupressure and pain control. I am sure that you will too. Be confident. Look to the future with assurance. Keep me informed of your progress. Drop me a line; I would love to hear from you. I will answer every letter.

This book covers many pain problems, but I admit this is by no means a complete list. If your problem is not discussed here, or you would like me to discuss your problem(s) with you, please feel free to consult me.

I welcome your help in organizing an acupressure workshop in your local area. Please contact my office concerning sponsorship. Whether you are a health care professional, a patient or a health enthusiast, I encourage you to participate so you can benefit from our unique workshops.

There are many aspects of Chinese medicine, such as The Chinese Way to Weight Control; Coping With Stress, The Chinese Way; Face Life; Chinese Herbal Medicine; Sex Secrets From China; Chinese Diet, etc.

If you are interested, please send $1.00 for a complete catalog to:

Dr. Pedro Chan
Center For Chinese Medicine
P.O. Box 478
Monterey Park, CA. 91754-0478

About the Author

Pedro Chan, Ph.D. is a nationally known health care educator and therapist, biomedical engineer, and Certified Acupuncturist (licensed by the State of California). He comes from a traditional Chinese medical family. His father is a doctor in Macao.

Dr. Chan's unique background has enabled him to evolve a new approach to the management and control of pain. Most of his patients have run the gamut of standard Western therapy and have failed to be relieved of their pain. Many of these patients who were told that their problems were "hopeless" and that they would have to "learn to live with pain," have gained pain control and find themselves free of pain, some after only a few treatments.

In the past few years, Dr. Chan has shared his knowledge with his colleagues, lecturing at many universities and medical centers. He has also personally trained (under the sponsorship of the Center for Chinese Medicine) thousands of medical and dental professionals across the country.

Currently, Dr. Chan is Director of the Chinese Total Health Center in Monterey Park, California. He has served as an Acupuncture Researcher for three years at White Memorial Medical Center, Los Angeles, and as an Acupuncture Examiner for the California State Board of Medical Quality Assurance. Dr. Chan has earned a Ph.D. in Biomedical Engineering. In 1975, he was honored with a Professorship by the Center For Health Education, Palos Verdes, California. In 1978, he was awarded a Doctorate of Philosophy in Oriental Medicine from the Institute of Oriental Medicine.

Dr. Chan is the author of many books and charts on various aspects of therapeutic Chinese medicine.

Other Price/Stern/Sloan books by Dr. Pedro Chan:

FINGER ACUPRESSURE
EAR ACUPRESSURE

Other works by Dr. Pedro Chan:

ACUPUNCTURE, ELECTRO-ACUPUNCTURE,
ANESTHESIA, *Borden Publishing Co., 1972*

WONDERS OF CHINESE ACUPUNCTURE
Borden Publishing Co., 1973

FINGER ACUPRESSURE, paperback edition,
Ballantine, 1975

ACUPUNCTURE MADE EASY (Co-translator)
Chan's Corp., 1975

ELECTRO-ACUPUNCTURE, ITS CLINICAL
APPLICATIONS IN THERAPY, *Chan's Corp., 1975*

EAR ACUPUNCTURE Wall Chart
Chan's Corp., 1973

HAND ACUPUNCTURE Wall Chart
Chan's Corp., 1973

ACUPUNCTURE NEWS (Editor)
Chan's Corp., 1974 - Present

THE CHINESE WAY TO WEIGHT CONTROL
Chan's Corp., 1980

DR. CHAN'S CHINESE DIET
Chan's Corp., 1980

THE FUTURE

"The doctor of the future will give no medicine, but will interest his patients in the care of the human frame, in diet, and in the care and prevention of disease."

–Thomas A. Edison